The information contained in Get Real! and Get Slim
for Life is not intended as a substitute for consulting
with your doctor or other healthcare provider. The
author has taken great care in the preparation of this
book, and has endeavoured to provide accurate, up to
date information, but does not warrant that the
information it contains will be free from errors or
omissions, or that it will be suitable for all readers'
purposes. The author and publisher are not
responsible for any adverse effects or consequences
resulting from the use of any suggestions, opinions, or
advice contained in this book. All matters relating to
your health should be discussed with your doctor.

ABOUT THE AUTHOR

Debbie Holden is a weightloss expert and the founder of Get Real! and Get Slim for Life, her multi-award winning programme that helps her clients to identify and address the real causes of their weight gain so that food no longer has the control it once did as well as working on releasing the excess weight.

Debbie and her Get Real! and Get Slim for Life Programme won the Best Weightloss Programme in the UK in November 2014 and were voted 'the best of the best'.

Described as an exceptional talent in the field of human potential, she is passionate about helping her clients achieve their goals.

Debbie has been a therapist in full-time private practice for almost 15 years and holds a Post Graduate Diploma in Hypnotherapy and Psychotherapy, A Masters Degree in Business and a BSc. (Hons.) degree in Psychology. She is also a Licensed Master Practitioner of NLP (Neuro-Linguistic

Programming), a Licensed Trainer of NLP and has qualifications in a variety of different therapies and techniques including EFT (Emotional Freedom Technique and Havening).

For more information about Debbie and her Programmes, go to:

www.debbieholden.com
www.facebook.com/GetSlimforLife

This book is dedicated to anyone who is tired of yo-yo dieting, anyone who is ready to try a different approach to releasing their excess weight and anyone who has decided NO MORE EXCUSES.

ACKNOWLEDGEMENTS

I would like to thank the thousands of amazing clients I have had the privilege of working with over the years, amazing people that have made me laugh, made me cry, and taught me so much about potential and the human mind. I am honoured to have been a part of their journey towards their goal weight.

A special heartfelt thanks goes to Kelly, Kim, Carol, Karen, Zoe and Val – a few of my amazing clients that have put their trust in me and allowed me test new ideas, therapies and techniques out on them over the years to help them achieve their goals – all without question!

To my family and friends – especially my mam and dad, my sister Vickie, my brother Sean and my best friend of 20 years, Jackie who have supported me throughout the years, rarely questioning even my most craziest of ideas and goals. I love you all.

GET REAL! AND GET SLIM FOR LIFE

I adore working with my clients, but because I work mainly on a one to one basis and as there are only so many hours in a day, it is impossible for me to help the amount of clients that want to work with me on a one to one basis.

I wrote this book in response to requests from women who, for a variety of reasons are unable to work with me personally. It is my wish that this book and my online programmes go some way towards bridging the gap.

The Get Real! and Get Slim for Life Programme is a two part process. One part contains all the tools and tips to help my clients release the excess weight. This is really the 'How To...' part of the Programme. It's this part of the Programme that helps people release the excess weight. The other part is therapy based and the goal here is to help my clients identify and address the real reasons behind their weight gain. It's this part of the Programme that helps them to keep the weight off over the long-term.

Whilst the therapy part of the Programme is tailored to each individual client, years of helping my clients achieve their goal weight showed that there were a number of elements that worked for every client, regardless of their starting weight and the information contained within this book is based on these elements.

The information you are about to read is exactly what I use with my VIP clients. Everything in this book has proved time and time again, that when applied consistently and persistently helps to not only release the excess weight but to keep it off long-term.

I have included the questions that I ask my clients so that you can work out what it is you really want and what has, until now, held you back from achieving your goal weight.

Releasing excess weight is simple, although at times, not always easy but if you apply the Principles of Get Real! And Get Slim for Life persistently and consistently, you will achieve the results you want.

The Get Real! And Get Slim for Life Programme is an alternative to dieting.

By applying the Principles consistently, you will find that you are able to regain the control you have handed over to food.

I believe that in order to reach your goal weight and then maintain it, traditional 'dieting' is neither necessary nor even desirable. By identifying and addressing the reasons for your weight gain amazing results can be achieved – all without dieting, weighing, counting or depriving yourself, however, you will need to make changes to your eating habits.

> **Remember:** persistence really does pay off and commitment to a goal ALWAYS results in the achievement of that goal. Without commitment NOTHING changes.

My experience of working with people who want to release their excess weight has shown that people fall into 2 categories:

- Those who are interested (in releasing their excess weight) and there are;
- Those who are committed (to releasing their excess weight).

A small girl, and her mum were sat in the garden playing and enjoying the sunshine. Their dog was sat nearby.

The dog was wriggling around and squirming and the little girl asked her mum why the dog was wriggling so much. Her mum replied, 'Don't worry about it'. The little girl wasn't satisfied with that as an answer and kept on asking why the dog was wriggling and squirming so much. Her mum eventually said, 'He's wriggling and squirming because he's sat on some nails'. 'Sat on some nails?' said the little girl. 'Why doesn't he just move?' Her mum replied…

'He's just not uncomfortable enough'.

Those who are interested in releasing their excess weight will do what is convenient, when it is convenient. They just aren't uncomfortable enough to stop sitting on the nails or committed enough to do what it takes to reach their goal weight.

Those who are committed to releasing their excess weight do whatever it takes to get to their goal, consistently and persistently and without excuses. They are uncomfortable enough to stop sitting on the nails and ready to do whatever it takes to reach their goal.

So, which are you?

Are you interested, or are you committed?

Remember:

You can have RESULTS
Or
You can have EXCUSES
YOU CAN'T HAVE BOTH

So, if you are committed to releasing the excess weight once and for all then you are about to enter a fabulous world of clever diet escapes. A world where you can expect real and lasting results.

Great things are
Not achieved by impulse
But by a series of small
Things brought together.
Vincent Van Gogh

INTRODUCTION

There are thousands of diets and ways of releasing excess weight around today, and even more books about the subject. It is my view that if diets actually worked long-term for most people who have signed up for them, there would only be a handful – but there aren't!

In the UK, in 2014 57% of women and 67% of men were classed as either overweight or obese (source: The Guardian, May, 2014), and with obesity levels continuing to rise, these figures will also continue to rise. The costs to the NHS of weight related issues stands at approximately £6 billion per year and this is also estimated to rise.

Today, the diet industry in the UK ONLY is worth more than £2 billion and yet, despite so much money being spent on diets, dieting and associated products, recent research conducted on behalf of The Telegraph showed that:

- 26% of women give up their latest diet within 7 days;
- 15% last 14 days;
- 31% last one month;
- 8% last 2 months, and
- 13% last between 3 and 6 months.

When explored in more detail, the reasons stated for giving up on reaching their goal weight included:

- Boredom
- Lack of willpower
- They had had a bad day (or in some cases, a good day)
- They spent all of their time thinking about everything they couldn't eat or drink
- They wanted a quick fix solution which really doesn't exist

After almost 15 years of working with my clients, I have heard all of these over the years, and a few more besides, BUT the major reason I have found for people not achieving their goal weight or quitting after a week or two is that...brace yourself...

FOOD HAS GOT LITTLE TO DO WITH IT

CHAPTER 1

Diets Don't Work!

But there again, I probably didn't need to tell you that!

There are so many adverts and posts on social media, etc., that guarantee amazing results just by taking a pill, a supplement, eating certain foods, not eating certain foods, drinking a bizarre mixture, etc. I'm sure you have seen some of them and some of you might also have signed up for them. I'm guessing that if you have signed up and bought them and you have still bought this book, they didn't deliver the miracles the adverts led you to believe you'd get.

Adverts like this lead to many people to having unrealistic expectations about what can actually be achieved in a short space of time. It's so easy to buy in to these claims when you are desperate for results but all they do is set you up for failure by leading you to have unrealistic expectations in the first place, not achieving the results they have promised and just giving up.

It's a similar story with diets. If they actually worked long term there would be a handful of them, instead of the thousands that are available.

Having unrealistic expectations of how YOUR body will respond will lead you to give up long before you reach your goal.

One of my clients released 4 ½ lbs of excess weight during the first week of working with me. To me, that was an amazing result, but my client didn't see it that way. She was devastated that she hadn't released the 7 lbs she had wanted to release. When I asked her if she has ever released 7 lbs in the first week of any weight release intervention she said no. See, what I mean about unrealistic expectations?

Fortunately she chose not to give up and we worked on putting her expectations into perspective and she has now released over a stone of excess weight in 9 weeks and has slimmed down by 13 inches.

Drastic results can and do happen when 'dieting' but what many don't realise is that it is water and not fat that has been released and this level of weightloss is impossible to maintain.

When a person has been on a low calorie or very low calorie diet, or has been cutting out or restricting food groups (cutting out or restricting food groups should only be done on the advice of a medical professional), the body goes into starvation mode so that when they start to eat 'normally' again, the body hangs on to what it receives in case it is deprived of fuel again. This means that they put the weight back on again (plus usually a bit more).

Each food group has vital nutrients that your body needs. Cutting out or restricting certain food groups is damaging to your body and messes up your metabolism.

Depending on your starting point (i.e. how much excess weight you have to release you might see fabulous results in the first couple of weeks but after that 1 – 2lbs per week is healthy and will take you towards your goal weight and then on to maintaining it over the long term.

To release the excess weight over the long term, you need to Get Real! About your expectations and apply ALL of the Principles consistently and persistently.

Remember: the weight didn't go on over night so it is not going to come off overnight, so this is a good place to re-visit your expectations so you don't set yourself up for failure.

When you get disheartened, think about the reasons that made you want to release the excess weight in the first place. (We'll cover this in more detail shortly).

Remember:

Diets only deal with what is on the **outside** (the excess weight), yet the triggers that have had you sprinting towards food when you weren't hungry or had you continuing to force food in even though you were already full are all on the **inside**.

When you identify and address what is going on inside your mind, food can no longer have the same control over you that it once had.
So, turn the page and let's get started on Getting Real! And Getting Slim for Life...

CHAPTER 2

PRINCIPLE 1

THE FANTASY BUBBLES THAT ARE KEEPING YOU STUCK

Time to Get Real!...Is it YOUR truth or THE truth?

What are fantasy bubbles? Fantasy bubbles are the stories that you've bought into; the stories or fantasies that you have told yourself so often that you now believe them.

BUT, just because you believe them, it doesn't make them true!

It simply means you've made them into YOUR truth – YOUR REALITY.

Here are some of the fantasy bubbles my clients have believed before they start working with me…

I'LL START ON MONDAY, NEXT WEEK, ON THE FIRST OF THE MONTH, AT NEW YEAR, AFTER MY HOLIDAY, ETC., ETC.

Many of my clients have described the lead up to the 'start date' as something along the lines of 'I'll eat as much as I can today and then I'll be good tomorrow…*really?!*

Time to Get Real!...The lead up to changing your life is NOT your last meal! Therefore, there is absolutely no need to binge. All this does is add to the amount of excess weight that needs to be released. Food is not scarce and, therefore, there is no reason to store it on your body for later.

I DON"T HAVE TIME

Time to Get Real!...make some! Refer back to 'are you interested in achieving your goal weight or are you committed to achieving it?'

I"LL BE HUNGRY

Time to Get Real!...Contrary to popular belief, feeling hungry is a GOOD thing! It tells you that your fuel tank needs topping up.

I CAN"T LOSE WEIGHT BECAUSE I'M ON MEDICATION

Time to get Real!...So are many of my clients and it hasn't stopped them.

EATING QUICKLY DOESN"T COUNT

Time to Get Real!...It so does! Eating quickly means you go from starving to stuffed without realising how you got there. You eat much more than you need, you possibly feel ill and there's probably a bit more excess weight to be released.

I HAVE AN UNDERACTIVE THYROID

Time to Get Real!...So do some slim people.

STANDING UP WHILE EATING DOESN'T COUNT

Time to Get real!...Oh yes it does!

I DON'T EAT ENOUGH AS IT IS SO I STRUGGLE TO LOSE THE EXTRA WEIGHT

Time to Get Real!...No one is fat in a famine.

I EAT HALF A PACKET OF BISCUITS AND TELL MYSELF I ONLY HAD TWO

Time to Get Real!...That's just delusional!

IF I EAT WHEN NO ONE IS THERE, IT DOESN'T COUNT

Time to Get Real!...It does. YOU are there and you do count.

LEAVING FOOD IS A WASTE

Time to Get Real!...And if you eat it, it will still end up as waste. If you have had enough and there's still food left, you are putting too much on your plate.

EATING IS THE ONE THING I CAN CONTROL

Time to Get Real!...Eating when you aren't hungry, continuing to eat after you have had enough or because you are tired, angry, fed up, because some one has upset you or because you are re-running old memories, etc. is NOT being in control.

FOOD IS MY FRIEND

Time to Get Real!...No it isn't! Food aside, I don't know anyone over the age of about 10 that has an inanimate object as a friend. Friends should uplift you, support you, encourage you and enhance your life because they are in it and because you are in theirs. Many of my clients have said that when they have eaten at those times they weren't hungry, they felt guilty, ashamed, a failure, etc. If my 'friends' made me feel like that, they wouldn't be my friends for long!

THAT PIECE OF CHEESECAKE, ETC. WAS CALLING TO ME

Time to Get Real!...No it wasn't! And if it was, there's probably more going on for you than just your weight...just saying!

IF YOU BREAK A BISCUIT OR A BAR OF CHOCOLATE INTO PIECES, THE CALORIES FALL OUT

Time to Get Real!...And, now we are back to being delusional!

I CAN'T BE BOTHERED

Time to Get Real!…OK, stay as you are!

Grab some and a pen (or pen and some paper if you don't want to write in your book) and make a list of all the fantasy bubbles you have made into your truth – your reality.

I'll eat as much as I can Today then
Start tomorrow
I have an underactive thyroid.
I work with food – picking is too easy
My Stomach is rumbling again.

Now, take each of your fantasy bubbles in turn and ask yourself:

Is it MY truth (my reality) or THE truth?

Remember: these are fantasy bubbles so there really is only one answer (and it isn't THE truth!)

Now imagine that each of these stories you've bought into are in a bubble…and just pop them. They aren't useful to you anymore and they certainly won't help you to achieve your goal weight.

So, did you identify your fantasy bubbles and pop them, or did you simply continue reading?

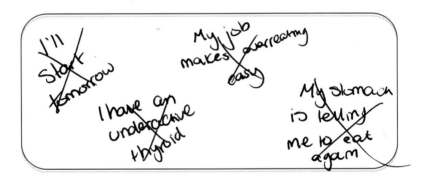

If you did identify and pop them – GREAT. Well done. You have started the process of getting out of your own way!

No? Why not? Remember – you can have results or excuses, you can't have both.

Regardless of the issue, whether it is over eating, drinking too much, etc. you do it because you get something out of it. For some of my clients, this is a difficult concept to get their head around. But, if they got nothing from it, they just wouldn't do it.

And also, you probably don't get from it what you think you get from it. What you get is a story you've bought into...another fantasy bubble.

Imagine you've had a bad day, you get home an think 'I could just do with a glass of wine to relax me'. You have it and then you buy into the story that now you're relaxed – you've created a new fantasy bubble. This is the problem – alcohol (or sugar, etc.) is a stimulant, not a relaxant but you've convinced yourself that wine relaxes you (2 + 2 = 5).

When you have another bad day, you (unconsciously) go to what you thought worked last time. At some point, one glass of wine, one biscuit, etc., isn't going to do it anymore so now you need two, then three, then four, etc., and what you thought of as a solution has now become a problem and has also probably resulted in even more excess weight.

This applies also to anything you are eating or drinking to manage your mood.

What original 'solutions' have now become problems for you?

I'll treat myself to chocolate because I'm not happy today.

I've not had much tea, crisps will make me feel better

I'll have a day off dieting. I was good yesterday

REMEMBER: POP THOSE BUBBLES EVERY TIME THEY COME UP

IT'S DO IT O'CLOCK

- Identify the fantasy bubbles that are keeping you stuck and POP them.

- Keep popping them whenever they come up.

- Decide once and for all 'NO MORE EXCUSES'.

CHAPTER 3

PRINCIPLE 2

IT'S ALL ABOUT YOU

Time to Get Real!...self-worth is all about you.

WHAT IS SELF-ESTEEM?

Self-esteem can be described as a person's overall sense of self-worth or personal value and can involve a variety of beliefs about ourself; self-judgements about our appearance, our beliefs, our emotions, our capabilities and our behaviours.

Although it can't be touched, your self-worth can affect how you feel.

Although it can't be heard, your self-worth is evident every time you talk about yourself, either to yourself or to others.

Although it can't be seen, your self-worth is there every time you look in a mirror.

IT'S ALL ABOUT YOU...WHY?

Your BELIEFS create your ATTITUDES

Your ATTITUDES create your THOUGHTS

Your THOUGHTS create your FEELINGS

Your FEELINGS create your DECISIONS

Your DECISIONS create your REALITY

WHAT DOES THIS MEAN IN TERMS OF YOUR WEIGHT?

Your BELIEFS create your ATTITUDES

This is where it all starts.

These are the things you believe and that you have turned into your attitudes about yourself since gaining weight. My clients have believed things such as 'I'm ugly', 'I'm huge', 'I hate myself', 'I've no willpower', 'I can't stick to anything', 'I'm useless', etc.

These types of phrases need eliminating from your vocabulary as soon as possible.

Imagine this: you get up in the morning, look in the mirror and start saying these types of things to yourself, then you expect to go out and have a great day. The likelihood of this great day happening after you have been so positive about yourself is pretty slim!

When you constantly repeat phrases like this to yourself, there is no way you will find the motivation to make the changes.

Remember the saying:

'If you can't say anything nice, don't say anything at all.'

Start practicing this often!

What things do you believe about yourself right now?

I'm fat
I'm ugly
I'm hard to love
I'm selfish
I'm disgusting

I have no willpower
I'll never be nappy
I'm huge
I have disgusting rolls
I have stretchmarks "

Your ATTITUDES create your THOUGHTS

Your attitudes create your day-to-day thoughts about your weight. For example, 'It's so hard to get rid of this weight', 'I'm in control of everything but this', 'Nothing ever works', 'I'll never get rid of this weight'. These then start to become self-fulfilling prophecies. For many, what then happens is that they then believe they won't achieve their goal weight and try half-heartedly or give up before they even start.

What are your day-to-day thoughts about your weight?

Its easier to give up
It comes off too slow
My goal weight is out of reach
3 Stone is a lot to lose
I can't stick to any diets long term

Your THOUGHTS create your FEELINGS

After thinking the thoughts, you start to feel bad about yourself, your weight, eating that biscuit, etc.

How do you feel about yourself, your weight, etc.?

I feel pathetic
I feel unhealthy
I feel like I can't control my eating habits
I feel ugly in my own skin

Your FEELINGS create your DECISIONS

When you aren't in a good place and you are feeling bad about yourself or your weight, many people head straight to the one thing that has made them unhappy – food. They head to the cake tin, the biscuit tin, the fridge, etc. They try to manage their mood by eating those things they think will cheer them up.

What do you do when you are feeling bad?

I fight with my own feelings
I secretly eat chocolate, chips etc
I tell myself it's all my fault
I stop moving and start moping around
I push people away

Your DECISIONS create your REALITY

That decision to eat because you are feeling bad will
result in you feeling worse, carrying more weight and
more importantly, reinforcing the beliefs and attitudes
that you identified as the starting point. And so the
cycle continues.

How does this affect you?

I get more and more depressed
I beat myself up.
My clothes start tearing at the seams
stomach hangs over my trousers
I give up AGAIN.

This applies to the negative outcomes of weight gain and, however, the opposite is also true.

Diets deal with your CURRENT REALITY, NOT with the reasons for your weight gain, which means that for many people, any results are short-term.

One of the first questions I ask each client that contacts me is 'What have you tried before?' Most of them reel off a list of diets, fitness regimes, etc. Many also tell them that one of them worked. My question is then 'So how can I help you?' Their answers are usually along the lines of 'Well, it worked while I did it'. I then ask 'So what happened for you to stop what was working and go back to unhelpful habits?' The answers usually include things like worry, tiredness, boredom, anxiety, stress, depression, etc.

This is crucial information, because unless these triggers are dealt with, the results achieved can only ever be short-term because as soon as those buttons are pressed, people ALWAYS go back to what they know – using food to change how they feel. This, as you know never lasts for very long. If food really did have the power to change how you feel, you would feel on top of the world – and those feelings would last for a long, long time, much longer than simply while you are eating.

There is also another issue here – food can NEVER EVER solve any problem other than genuine, physical hunger. This means that what ever it was that caused you to turn to food is still going to be there after you have finished eating. It's still going to need to be dealt with, along with even more weight to shift.

So it makes sense that if you only deal with the excess weight, the results will be short-term.

To achieve your goal and maintain it over the long-term you need to identify your triggers and address them so that food does not have the control it had in the past.

It is in your

moments

of decisions

that your destiny

is shaped

Tony Robbins

You need to do something different. Doing more of
the same means you get more of the same.

Or...

If you do what you've always done,

you'll get what you've always gotten.

And if that didn't bring it home to you, then...

The definition of insanity is doing the

same thing over and over again and expecting

different results.

Albert Einstein

Instead of focusing on old problems, we need to turn
our mind to creating new solutions.

Keep up with the beliefs and attitudes you currently have and your reality WILL STAY THE SAME.

Change your beliefs and attitudes and your reality WILL change.

Remember: problems cannot be solved at the level at which they were created, so if you continue to use food to change how you feel, you won't ever reach your goal.

Your BELIEFS create your ATTITUDES

How will your beliefs and attitudes change about
yourself as you Get Real!?

I will believe I can achieve my goals
I am not worthless on the inside or outside
I will learn to love myself
I will change my negative attitude to a
positive one.

Your FEELINGS create your DECISIONS

What decisions WILL you make going forward?

I will stop relying on chocolate fixes
I will be patient with my weight loss
I will look at how far I have come, instead
of how far I have to go.
I will change my attitude towards food

Your DECISIONS create your REALITY

What will your NEW reality be as you Get Real!?

> I will be happy in my own skin
> Healthy eating will NOT be a chore
> I will not give in to bad foods
> because of a bad/sad mood.
> I won't keep blaming myself for everything

We live in a quick fix society. There are pills to help people stop smoking, pills to change how people feel, pills to reduce anxiety and there are pills to help people release excess weight.

In many cases, these are treated as little more than sticking plasters. Unless the person is prepared to do their bit as well as taking the medication, it isn't going to make much difference. For example, if a person takes tablets to help them stop smoking and then decide that they'll 'just have one, just to see', many of them will go back to smoking.

43

I have worked with clients who have been prescribed diet pills by their doctor – the type that restricts the amount of fat that can be absorbed into the body. On the face of it, it seems like one answer to the problem, yet many of the clients I've worked with who were prescribed these tablets didn't see them as a way of helping them to reach their goal. They saw them as permission to eat more fat.

Other clients who, in the past, attended some of the well known 'turn up once a week and get weighed' diet plans have told me that there is now a period of time (6 weeks, I believe) that they can have off the plan – they don't need to attend the weigh-in and there are no consequences to missing these weeks. Did they see these weeks as weeks where they could attend special events or go on holiday, etc.? No! They saw them as opportunities to binge.

WHERE DO YOU START?

You start by accepting yourself and your situation as it is now. Until you can accept yourself AND all of your imperfections, little will change. Accepting yourself does not mean you have to like what you see, but it does mean that you can work on your goals without sabotaging yourself.

Accepting yourself means:

- Taking complete responsibility for where you are and where you want to be.
- Getting out of denial.
- Knowing your starting point.
- Making the decision that achieving your goal weight is a major priority in your life and following through with consistent action.

If you are going to focus on weighing yourself all the time to see if you've shed a pound or gained a pound, then the chances are you are doomed for failure. The emotional effects of constantly weighing yourself can be devastating. So beware of the scales – they can turn into your enemy. Scales are just ONE measuring tool – not the only one. The scales don't control your weight but they can definitely control the way you see yourself.

One of my clients was retaining fluid during her time of the month and that week the scales showed an increase in weight of 3 lbs. She also measured herself. Even though the scales didn't show her what she wanted to see, the tape measure did. She had still shrunk by 3 inches.

TAKING COMPLETE RESPONSIBILITY FOR WHERE YOU ARE NOW AND FOR WHERE YOU WANT TO BE

Your mission here is to start to break free from the self-imposed prison you have built around yourself. Taking complete responsibility for where you are now means it's time to turn the excuses you have turned into reasons for not yet achieving your goal weight back into excuses.

Acknowledge that whatever 'reasons' you have used for not achieving your goal, are in fact excuses. Decide once and for all 'NO MORE EXCUSES'.

For your reality to change, you need to admit to yourself that it is YOU and ONLY YOU that has got you to a place where you are unhappy with your weight. Whatever the triggers were, it was YOU that put food into your mouth when you weren't hungry and it was YOU that continued to eat despite having had enough. No one was stood pointing a gun at your head while they forced you to eat!

Stepping up and taking responsibility for your current reality can be difficult but taking responsibility is the only way things are going to change.

Blaming work, your childhood, the dog, the kids, Coronation Street, etc., is not taking responsibility – it's being in denial. Whilst these types of things might contribute to how you feel, it is you who has chosen to hang on to them and then to use food to blot them out, stuff them down or change how you feel about them.

Remember:

You can't reach for anything new if your hands are still full of yesterday's junk.

Are you prepared to take full responsibility for where you are now?

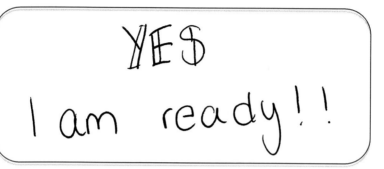

(There are three possible answers to this question – Yes, No and I'll try).

YES?

Congratulations! You are on your way towards sorting out your weight once and for all.

NO?

Thank you for your honesty, but be aware that until you are prepared to take full responsibility NOTHING is going to change for you.

I'll TRY

No you won't! When we say 'I'll try', what we are doing is seeking approval for something we know we aren't going to do. We are simply giving ourself permission to fail.

Decide to either do it or decide not to do it – these are the only real choices. If you choose not to do it, there is little point in reading any further. If however, you choose to take responsibility then congratulations! You will soon be getting real and getting slim for life.

If you are ready to Get Real! and Get Slim fro Life, you need to know your starting point – so GET WEIGHED.

The next thing to do is to take complete responsibility for where you want to be. Know this – YOU are in control of both your weight and your results. Nothing and no one else – it's all down to you. So, decide now that you will do whatever it takes to reach your goal weight. This means among other things, identifying and dealing with the issues that have sent you sprinting towards food instead of towards your goal weight.

**Decide now to make yourself and your results a
priority in your life.**

What is your current weight?

12 stone & 4 pounds

What is your goal weight?

8 stone & 7 pounds

What is your goal behind your goal weight?

To identify your goal behind your goal ask yourself the following questions:
What will be different about your life when you are at your goal weight?
What will be in your life that you don't have now?
What will you do or have that you don't do or have now?

I won't lose my breath though simple activities
I won't have to worry how I look
I will be happy to get 'dressed up'

I will have the confidence that I don't have now
I won't worry what people are saying about my body
My heart will be healthier.
It will be easier to love myself

Please be patient. Reducing your weight properly and safely takes time. Many people expect to release lots of weight in a few weeks despite them taking years to put it all on. That's unrealistic isn't it?

What you think about is what you get in life. We tend to get what we pay most attention to. So if you pay attention to the positive things that are happening to you, you'll get more of them. If you focus on what stays the same, things stay the same. Whether you are experiencing small changes or big changes doesn't matter – what matters is that changes are happening. Think back to my client who was disappointed with a 3 lb gain because she was retaining fluid – if she had focused on that she would probably have just given up. Instead she chose to focus on the inches she'd shrunk.

Your subconscious (autopilot) mind works non stop, 24 hours a day, 7 days a week regardless of whether you are awake or asleep and together with your conscious (thinking) mind, a unique partnership is created.

Think of your mind like a ship. Your conscious (thinking) mind is the captain and has responsibility for setting the direction of the ship and giving the orders. Your subconscious (autopilot) mind is the crew that carry out the captains commands.

The main way that the captain communicates with the crew is through thoughts. Every thought is a command for your subconscious mind to obey. The commands you repeat most often and those connected to the strongest emotions become the commands that your subconscious mind obeys.

Remember: our brains like things ahead of us to aim at and the closer they are, the better. That is why often the goal of chocolate in the next few minutes seems more desirable than getting into a certain outfit in 3 months time. If getting into a particular outfit is your goal, make sure you have plenty of smaller goals built in along the way.

DENIAL

Denial keeps you stuck. Before starting Get Real! and Get Slim for Life, many of my clients would only look in a mirror that was big enough only for them to see their head and shoulders. Full length mirrors and shop windows were avoided like the plague. Remember – unless you know exactly where you are now and what you are dealing with – you are in denial.

Some people also try to convince themselves that the things they are missing out on because of their weight aren't really that important. If you feel like you are missing out on things, yet put them to the back of your mind or pretend they don't matter, you are in denial and you are back into excuses.

If you have no idea of how much you weigh, you are in major denial. If you don't have an accurate understanding of where you are now, how will you know how much weight to release to reach a healthy weight and more importantly, how will you know when you get there?

If you don't know your starting point, there is a danger that you will start to blame anything and everything for your situation (for example, blaming retailers for clothes sizes getting smaller, blaming the washer or the dryer for clothes shrinking, etc!)

Remember: denial can take many forms. Not knowing your starting point is only one of them. Here are some other ways of being in denial:

- You get weighed and the scales stay the same as they were last week or you've put on a pound or two. You tell yourself and any one who will listen that you've done everything you were supposed to do and you've no idea what's happened…Really?!

- You convince yourself that a cream cake, a glass of wine, a family sized bag of sweets (or two) won't really make much difference …Really?!

- You convince yourself that when out for a meal it would be rude not to eat everything put in front of you...Really?!

Knowing your staring point is essential. YOU NEED TO GET WEIGHED. The best time to do this is on the same day each week, first thing in the morning as soon as you get up, have been to the toilet and before getting dressed and eating or drinking anything. This will give you the most accurate reading to chart your progress.

If you don't have any scales and decide to get weighed while you are out shopping, remember that to chart your progress accurately, you need to go at the same time, wearing exactly the same clothes and making sure you have eaten and drunk exactly the same things each time.

For many, their self-worth can be wrapped up in what the scales say. If you obsess over the scales, STOP IT! Remember, they are only one tool.

Remember:

SCALES

DO NOT MEASURE YOUR SELF-WORTH

One of my clients was asked to get weighed ONLY on the morning of each session. She didn't. What she did was get weighed four days after the first session. She had released 7 lbs (half a stone).

Understandably, she was over the moon, but this soon turned to devastation when she got weighed three days later on the morning of her next session. The scales hadn't moved – she was still only 7 lbs lighter. She started to beat herself up, questioned whether or not it was working (OK!), whether it was worth it, etc. All of a sudden, something that was to be celebrated (releasing 7 lbs in a week without dieting) became, in her mind a failure.

DON'T SABOTAGE YOUR OWN SUCCESS LIKE THIS

Another way to chart your progress is to measure yourself every week. Measure the key areas – upper arms, chest, waist, hips and thighs and make a note of these each week. The weeks that you don't see a difference on the scales for, for example time of the month, etc., can still show a difference in measurements.

Another way is to choose a piece of clothing from your wardrobe. What you are looking for is a piece of clothing that you could wear if you had to but that would dig in after a while and become uncomfortable. Try it on after getting weighed each week (or instead of getting weighed) so you know how it feels. It will soon become comfortable and when it does, simply choose something else that you could wear if you had to. Keep repeating this process until you are at your goal weight. Don't choose something you can't get into at all because your motivation will go downhill and you will reinforce your beliefs and attitudes about your weight.

As you release the excess weight and clothes become too big, GET RID OF THEM. If you want to keep a reminder of how far you have come, then keep ONE item of clothing and use this only as a reminder of your success since taking responsibility and action. Keeping clothes that are too big is giving yourself permission to slip back into old habits.

Have you got weighed yet?

What is your starting point?

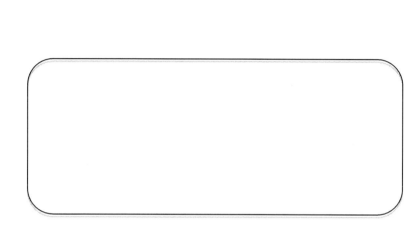

Get weighed, measured and/or choose a piece of clothing to help you monitor your progress.

Remember: it is better to hurt for half an hour than to be in denial for a few more years.

In any moment of decision, the best thing you can do is the right thing, the next best thing you can do is the wrong thing and the worst thing you can do is nothing.
Theodore Roosevelt

Remember: Your world reflects back to you YOUR beliefs.

Wanting or expecting your world to change without doing anything to change it, is like looking in a mirror and expecting the reflection to smile back first.

In other words, if you expect results without putting in any effort to get them, reaching your goal weight simply isn't going to happen (refer back to Einstein's quote about insanity!)

IDENTIFING YOUR TRIGGERS

Over the next few weeks, keep a note of what is happening at those times you feel compelled to eat even though you aren't hungry. BUT instead of going straight for food, decide what it is you really want and do that instead.

So, if you are tired, rest. If you are bored, do something that you enjoy that doesn't involve food or catch up on some jobs that need doing. If you are fed up, phone a friend.

Remember, these are the times when you need to make YOU and your goal a priority - NOT food. Also remember that if you do make food the priority instead of You, you will still be tired, bored, fed-up, etc. after you have eaten, probably more so because now you have just sabotaged your success.

This is the key element of the work I do with my clients. Once you have identified your triggers, think of ways of dealing with them that don't involve food.

What are the triggers that send you to food at times you are not physically hungry?

feeling down   Lack of focus
Lack of sleep
Boredom
Thinking about food

What can you do instead that will deal more effectively with these triggers and yet, don't involve food?

> Listen to music
> play Scrabble
> colour in.
> Read dog training tips
> Plan finances

If you are struggling to address the triggers fully, consider seeking therapy to help you.

Remember: Eating or drinking to change how you feel is emotional eating.

We'll cover this in more detail later.

Remember:

It's all about YOU. Time to change IMPOSSIBLE to I'M POSSIBLE.

IT'S DO IT O'CLOCK

- Take responsibility for where you are now.

- Get weighed so you know your starting point.

- Work out where you want to be and realistic timescales to get there.

- Make yourself and your goal a priority in your life.

- Stop making excuses.

- As you drop dress sizes, get rid of any clothes that are too big.

- Identify the triggers that have you eating when you are not physically hungry.

- When these triggers are fired, do something that deals with the triggers (and that doesn't involve food).

- If necessary, seek professional help to assist you in addressing your triggers.

CHAPTER 4

PRINCIPLE 3

UNDERSTANDING HUNGER

Time to Get Real!...food has absolutely no impact on hunger of the mind.

Calorie counting, weighing, measuring, horrible tasting food supplements, pills, etc., that come with 'dieting' are never going to create permanent weight release because:

The body treats dieting like a famine so as soon as you come off one, the body goes into overdrive, hoarding calories as fat in readiness for the next time. It also slows down your metabolism so you burn fewer calories. These are some of the reasons that yo-yo dieting makes you heavier.

Of course, diets often achieve short-term results but keeping the excess weight off requires you do something different.

Making changes both on the inside (addressing and dealing with your triggers) and the outside (following the Principles of Get Real! and Get Slim for Life consistently) will give you long term results.

Food has become something it was never intended to become. In the past food was nothing more that the sustenance needed to get us through the day; to provide our bodies with the fuel and energy it needed to work, think and play. Today, food has become something very different. It's something many turn to when they are happy, sad, angry, frustrated, tired, bored, etc. – it's become mood management.

Before setting off on a long journey many of us will fill the fuel tank so we have enough fuel for at least a good part of the journey. So with a full tank we are driving along happily for a while and then the oil light comes on.

Putting more fuel in the tank isn't going to deal with the issue of the oil, yet many people with an issue with their weight rarely, if ever consider this. They eat and then a little while later they have an argument, get stuck in traffic, are tired, fed-up or bored etc., and rather than deal with the issue, they put more fuel in the tank.

The issue is still there and now there's too much fuel in the tank.

When food becomes no more than fuel, you think about it when your fuel tank needs topping up – you don't think about it before the oil light comes on.

When your car is parked on the drive or in the garage, can you honestly say you spend that much time thinking about it? No.

You think about it when you are about to go out, when it needs cleaning or when you need fuel, etc., so why would you constantly think about the one thing (food) that has got you to a place where you are unhappy before you need to re-fuel?

There are two types of hunger:

Hunger of the body (physical hunger)

This is when your fuel tank is empty and needs topping up. This is usually when you need to eat (remember: it's easy to confuse hunger with thirst, but we'll cover this shortly).

Physical hunger:

- Builds gradually
- Starts in the stomach
- Occurs several hours after a meal
- Goes away when you have eaten

Hunger of the mind (emotional hunger)

This is everything else and happens when you turn to food to change how you feel.

Emotional hunger:

- Develops suddenly
- Starts above the neck (thoughts)
- Is unrelated to the time since you last ate
- Leads to more emotions (guilt, anger at self, frustration at sabotaging your success, etc.)
- Persists despite not being physically hungry

Hunger of the mind persists despite you not being physically hungry. One of my clients once explained that it didn't matter how much she ate she never felt full. On the one hand, to never feel full is impossible, yet on the other hand it's completely possible. To explain...however much a person has stretched their stomach through over eating, it can only hold so much, therefore to never feel full is impossible.

Food can ONLY EVER satisfy physical hunger; it can never fill an emotional gap. So if you have been using food to deal with emotional situations you will never feel full simply because you eating isn't going to make any difference to the situation that compelled you to eat.

Recognising what you are feeling is essential if you eat at any time other than when you are not genuinely, physically hungry.

Ask yourself 'What am I feeling?' And then be honest with yourself. If it is genuine hunger – eat. If it is emotional hunger – deal with what is really going on.

Dealing with these feelings is a powerful tool that will stop you from self-medicating with food. Remember, whatever caused the feelings will still be there when you stop eating.

Think of this: if someone treats you badly, what happens? They walk away and forget all about it. What do you do? You probably keep replaying it over and over and over again. You start talking to yourself about it over and over and over again. And then what do you do? You probably go and find something to eat to change how you feel and then beat yourself up for eating because now you feel as bad as you did when you were replaying the situation. And guess what...eating hasn't changed the actual situation and now you feel just as bad, if not more so.

Just let it go...BEFORE you start replaying it. If you replay it over and over and over again and then make yourself feel bad because you've eaten something in order to change how you feel, you are only punishing yourself for their behaviour. The ONLY person that is being punished is YOU by YOU. Why would you punish yourself for someone else's behaviour. Doing this regularly has probably contributed to your weight being at a level you are unhappy with.

WHAT IS EMOTIONAL EATING?

Emotional eating means eating in response to particular feelings such as stress, boredom, tiredness, etc.

Emotional eating patterns are based on unconscious beliefs that eating at these times brings a positive emotional benefit (e.g. comfort) and the urge to eat is not about food itself. It's based on a strong unconscious need to feel the feeling that you associate with it.

The key to overcoming emotional eating is to become aware of the unconscious patterns and beliefs that underpin the problem and then work to change them.

FOOD AND LOVE

For many, food equates to love – it's unavoidable. When a baby feels hunger – it doesn't know what this is, it just feels uncomfortable. The baby is then fed and feels better and so, right from the early days, a link between being loved and being fed is created. It also works the other way too. The care giver is expressing love by offering milk or food, etc. to the baby.

One problem with this connection however, is that it can lead to those wanting to show love doing so by pushing food onto people and creating a pressure on them to eat inappropriately (e.g. too much in terms of portion size, cake or a snack when they are not hungry, etc). By saying 'NO' it might be perceived as rejection BUT:

Remember: When you say YES to someone else, make sure that you are not saying NO to yourself.

Before you say YES, remind yourself of all the reasons you are doing this Programme (your goals behind your goals).

COMFORT

Due to the connection between food and love, food is often used as a means of giving comfort. This also very often starts in childhood and creates a link in the child's mind which can easily continue into adulthood. Occasionally, there is nothing wrong with this, but if this is the process every evening while watching TV, or when you want to change how you feel, it becomes a problem.

Not only does food bring comfort because of the link with love, it can also create a chemical high. This then affects your metabolism and causes your blood sugars to spike and you experience a sugar rush. Your brain counters this by increasing the amounts of serotonin and melatonin in your system (2 chemicals which are known to cause drowsiness). Cue: sugar rush.

The first step in addressing your emotional eating is to establish a good understanding of what is really going on when you are drawn to eat when you are not hungry.

Earlier I asked you to write down your goal and the goals behind your goal. I'm going to ask you now to consider the goals behind the goals in relation to emotional eating.

For example, there is a deadline looming at work and you know you are going to struggle to meet it, your stress levels are rising and you just need sugar! Your goal is to eat. Your goal behind your goal is to relieve the stress you are feeling. However, relieving the stress you are feeling is only going to occur while you are eating. The deadline is still there and now you've just wasted time eating when you could have been getting on with what you needed to do.

When I eat emotionally it is to take my mind off the troubles I am facing. A problem at work or dealing with grief. I can forget while I'm eating

When you emotionally eat, what is your goal behind the goal to eat? What are you trying to change? You will need to consider this for all situations that compel you to eat to manage your feelings.

Completing a food diary will help you to identify when you are emotionally eating. It's also a good idea to make a note of the feeling that made you want to eat at that time. It can also be helpful to make a note of exactly what was going on at the time that caused you to feel this way.

Ask yourself:

- When I get the urge to eat, what is it I really want?
- If there was something I believed I was getting from eating at this time (that isn't to do with hunger), what might it be?
- To what extent does eating at this time really provide that emotional benefit (be honest)?

As you look at your food diary, you may notice patterns emerging that will help you to identify triggers for emotionally eating (people, places, certain times, etc). Try to change as many of these triggers as possible in order to interrupt the thought processes, for example, make small changes to your routine – sit in a different chair to watch TV, plan to do different activities to occupy your mind at those times you experience the urge to emotionally eat, develop a plan to deal with what is really going on.

Now take a look at the feelings that currently have you reaching for food when you are not hungry and think about what you really want from it. Does it really relax you? Does it really alleviate boredom? Or...does it just seem that way?

There are bound to be far more effective ways of feeling the feeling you want to experience, so take some time to really think about what you could be doing instead to create those particular emotional benefits that you are craving.

This is about prioritising your own well being and challenging the way you usually approach eating, so think beyond those things which immediately come to mind.

As you change your habits and deliberately create those feelings that you usually look for from food, your belief that you need to eat in order to experience them will fade.

Remember:

You can't start the next chapter of your life while you are still re-reading the last one.

Also remember:

Food has absolutely no impact on hunger of the mind.

IT'S DO IT O'CLOCK

- Separate hunger of the body from hunger of the mind.

- When you are physically hungry - eat.

- When you are emotionally hungry, deal with the real issue.

- Remind yourself of what is important – reaching your goal weight or that piece of cake, etc. The time that cake becomes more important than your health and well being is the time you really need to start dealing with the real reasons behind your weight gain.

CHAPTER 5

PRINCIPLE 4

FUEL – THE 4-LETTER WORD OF WEIGHTLOSS

Time to Get Real!...Food is NOTHING more than FUEL.

Now you know your starting point, your goal and you have identified your triggers and hopefully you have started to address them.

Look at the following examples of food and drink. Which would you say are good and bad when it comes to releasing excess weight?

✓ Salad	✗ Chocolate	⅃ Bread	✗ Wine
✓ Water	✗ Chips	✗ Cake	✗ Donut
✓ Fruit	⅃ Fizzy drinks	✗ Crisps	✗ Take away

The fact is none of them are either good or bad...

When you stop classifying foods and drinks as either good or bad, you get rid of the desire to binge. If you KNOW YOU CAN HAVE IT you stop obsessing about it.

The Get Real! and Get Slim for Life Programme is not a diet. Start to see food as nothing more than fuel rather than as something to manage your moods and you will eat when you are physically hungry instead of when you are emotionally hungry and the excess weight has no option but to melt away.

Remember:

Food is nothing more than fuel

IT'S DO IT O'CLOCK

- Eat food only when you need re-fuelling.

- Don't deprive yourself of anything but eat only when you are physically hungry.

CHAPTER 6

PRINCIPLE 5

MANAGING YOUR APPETITE

Time to Get real!...size IS important!

There are many reasons people overeat, for example:

- Continual grazing means that the feeling of being hungry or the feeling of being satisfied is less likely to occur.

- The over-processing of food means that it is easier to eat and feeling satisfied is less likely or it takes much more food to feel satisfied.

- Some people believe that they are depriving themselves if they don't eat a huge plateful of food or finish that has been served to them.

- Some see it as a sign of weakness to leave food.

- Many are brought up to believe it is wrong not to eat everything on their plate.

- Many people eat unconsciously.

- Old programming – I have had many clients who were brought up with little food available and they were in effect programmed that if there is food there, it should be eaten because it might not be there tomorrow.

- Society rules, e.g. It's Christmas, overeat, It's Easter, eat as much chocolate as you can, You're on holiday, eat and drink more than you do at home, it's an all you can eat buffet and you want your moneys worth.

- Remember: all you can eat is NOT a challenge!

HOW WELL DO YOU KNOW YOUR FAT?

Did you know:

- Your fat cell cells can grow up to 1000 times their original size.
- Once a fat cell has reached its maximum capacity your body will produce a new fat cell to store the additional fat in.
- Once a new fat cell has been formed it is yours to keep. You can't get rid of it. All you can do is reduce its size.

We all have a number of fat cells in our body. During the last three months of pregnancy, fat cells are formed in the developing foetus and again at the start of puberty when hormones start to kick in. After puberty the body doesn't normally produce new fat cells, they simply get bigger and bigger as the body stores more fat. One exception to this is if an adult gains a significant amount of weight. In order to store the additional fat the body forms new fat cells. So, when your weight increases, these fat cells expand and when you reduce your weight, they shrink.

Non obese adults have approximately 30-50 billion fat cells, however, obese adults have approximately 60 – 100 billion.

Fat tissue is made up of fat cells and can be thought of as tiny bags that each hold a drop of fat. When you eat a meal or a sugary snack, enzymes break the fats down into fatty acids. These fatty acids are then absorbed from the blood into fat cells, muscle cells and liver cells. Once in these cells, through the stimulation of insulin, the fatty acids are turned into fat molecules and are stored as fat droplets.

The body is 10 times more efficient at simply storing fat in a fat cell than it is at converting protein and carbohydrates into fat. Given a choice, a fat cell will grab the fat and store it rather than the carbohydrates or protein because it's a much easier process for the body to carry out.

Fat leaves the body through sweat, by breathing out carbon dioxide and contrary to popular belief, through urine. So the more you drink and the purer the fluid you drink, the faster your fat leaves your body and the faster your fat cells shrink.

HUNGER V THIRST

The feelings for hunger and thirst are exactly the same. What tends to happen is that we get THAT feeling and automatically think 'I need food' when what we probably need is fluid.

Increasing your water intake has many benefits: it hydrates you; it flushes out your system and it prevents you eating when you are actually thirsty. The purer the fluid, the quicker and easier it is to flush out your system.

You'll probably end up going to the toilet more, but rather than see it as a nuisance or as an inconvenience, see it instead as getting rid of a bit more fat!

HOW TO DRINK

For a few decades now we have been encouraged to drink little and often, however, this can lead to dehydration because drinking little and often means our cells are unable to collect sufficient fluid to hydrate us. It can also be very easy to lose our sense of thirst by drinking little and often which leads to confusion between the signals for thirst and hunger. When our cells become dehydrated they go into survival mode and store fat (this then becomes a source of energy for use when we need it). When they are in survival mode, our cells get rid of the water and retain the fat. By drinking little and often (not enough in one go to hydrate our cells), we store fat.

Think of it this way:

Drinking little and often is similar to putting a bit of water on a sponge. This isn't going to get the sponge wet and during the time in between topping up, it is likely to evaporate.

Soaking the sponge with sufficient water means that it gets completely hydrated. Drinking a glass or two of water (depending on your thirst) in one go will hydrate your cells fully.

Once hydrated, drink when you are thirsty. Children do this very well. They run around for a while and then stop for a drink. They drink until their thirst is satisfied and then they go back to what they were doing. Our brain will switch off the 'thirsty feeling' when we are about 80% hydrated to stop us from drinking too much.

If this doesn't convince you to drink more water think about this – for every litre of water our body loses, we compensate with 1 kg (2.2lbs) of fat.

WHAT ABOUT SUGARY DRINKS?

There are two problems with drinking sugary drinks. Firstly they contain calories and therefore, will impact on your results. Secondly and perhaps more importantly, the brain does not understand that these types of drinks are liquids and therefore treats them as food which can then get the fat storage tanks going once again.

Artificially sweetened drinks can also impact on your results. The taste of artificial sweeteners is about 200 times sweeter than sugar, but without the calories. The brain expects these calories and realises it hasn't had them so it increases the appetite in order to get what it expects.

So in order to stay hydrated, stick to water, herbal teas (without sugar or sweetener), or sugar/sweetener/calorie free drinks. Once hydrated, tea and coffee are fine but make sure you stay hydrated by drinking when you are thirsty and drinking until your thirst has been satisfied.

Rather than eat when you get THAT feeling, drink a large glass of water instead, wait 20 minutes and the chances are the feeling of hunger will go away. If the feeling doesn't go away, make sure it is physical hunger and not emotional hunger you are feeling. If it is physical hunger – re-fuel. If it's emotional hunger – deal with the real issue.

WHAT ABOUT ALCOHOL?

Alcohol can hinder your results as it stimulates your appetite. Whilst you might feel satisfied from a meal, a comparable amount of calories from several drinks won't satisfy you in the same way. Alcohol is high in calories so reducing the amount you drink will help you towards your goal. Alcohol can also affect your willpower so it is likely you might overeat. To avoid this, alternate every drink with a glass of water or other low calorie/low sugar drink (or a calorie/sugar free drink).

A bottle of wine is packed with sugar and toxins – poisonous substances which can be harmful if done over and over again and which can cause hangovers.

Red wine has more toxins than white wine but beware, white wine contains more sugar than red wine – up to 4 tablespoons per bottle. Even dry wines have a high sugar content. Champagne and sweet dessert wines can have as much as ½ a pound of sugar per litre.

PLATE SIZE AND PORTION SIZE

Plates have got bigger and bigger and bigger.

Think about it…we break a plate or two and at some point we decide to buy a new set. We go to the shop, put them in the trolley and when we get home, at some point they go in the cupboard.

How many times do you actually check to see if the new plates are the same size as the ones already in the cupboard? How often do you consider where in the pile of plates they fit? What tends to happen is that they go in the cupboard, usually underneath the others, they get taken out, piled up with food without thinking about whether they contain the same amount of food as used to be put on the old plates and then we wonder why in a short space of time, clothes have got tighter.

Even if you do get real about this and don't fill the new larger plate, it rarely works. When there is more plate than portion, the brain says 'nice try'! Use a smaller plate and you will feel satisfied. Why? Because the dish is full.

WHAT SIZE PLATE SHOULD YOU BE USING?

One that has a diameter of no more than 18 cm or 7 inches, excluding the lip.

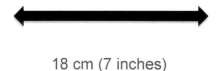

18 cm (7 inches)

Amazon, as well as other retailers have a good selection of healthy portion plates that are the correct size.

PORTION SIZE

Portions, as well as plates have also got much bigger. Just think about going to a restaurant or a pub. You order a meal and what turns up is the equivalent of a trough. So what do you do? There's a really good chance that you tell yourself that you've paid for it so you are going to eat it. Then you FORCE it all down until you feel ill. You force it down because you have paid for it, or for any other story you have bought into.

So how much has forcing down that food actually cost you? Obviously, there's the cost of the meal, but what is rarely thought about are all of the other costs (you feel ill, the button on your trousers is now marking your skin and there's a really good chance that you have just increased your weight). There are also the emotional costs, for example, now you are beating yourself up, feeling that you have let yourself down, angry with yourself, etc.

Was it REALLY worth it? If you had already had enough to eat when you continued to force down what was left, did you REALLY enjoy it?

Remember: a portion of food is roughly the SIZE OF YOUR FIST and should be a layer and not a mountain! Eating until you are full (rather than eating until you are satisfied) is OVEREATING.

One of my clients had no problem stopping eating as soon as she was satisfied and leaving whatever was left when she was at home. But she had a real problem doing this when eating out. It wasn't that she decided that she was paying for it so she was going to eat it, it was because she felt embarrassed that someone had cooked it and felt obliged to eat it.

Remember: if you are paying for it, you choose how much of it to eat! Don't let other people or situations sabotage your goals or your results. This also applies when eating with family or friends. If you don't want to offend them and you don't want to sabotage your results, warn them in advance that you are cutting down your portion sizes.

Remember: When you say YES to someone or something, make sure you are not saying NO to yourself.

WHAT ABOUT PUDDING?

Remember this is NOT a diet so puddings are good - as a TREAT! But – instead of forcing it in on top of everything else, leave a pudding size amount of food on your plate from the previous course. If you are having a treat, make sure that it is really a treat and enjoy it rather than stuffing it in on top of everything else, not taste it and not even enjoy it that much.

ARE YOU A MEMBER OF THE CLEAN PLATE CLUB?

Were you brought up to eat everything on your plate? Do you now find it difficult to leave food, even when you have had enough?

Remember: being told to clear your plate was appropriate when it was being said – you are now an adult and you have choices. You can make a different decision.

Get into the habit of leaving some food on your plate. This sends a signal to your unconscious mind that food is not scarce.

If you are still uncomfortable leaving food on your plate, PUT LESS ON IT IN THE FIRST PLACE!

Remember: Only ever eat for flavour – NEVER for quantity.

WASTE

Remember, waste is waste so whether you eat it or leave it, it will end up as waste. The decision YOU must make is whether you want it IN THE WASTE or ON YOUR WAIST.

TREATS

A further problem is that eating between meals is often seen as having a treat. Again, this is often set in motion during childhood. Children are given treats if they have been good or in some way 'deserve them'. The availability of food now means that treating yourself is a very easy thing to do. Treats, by definition are designed to be occasional! Re-allocating them back to occasional allows you to take back control.

NUTRITIONAL ADVICE

Whilst Get Real! and Get Slim for Life is not a diet, in order for you to shed your excess weight some changes will be required, for instance:

- Eat less fat
- Eat less sugar
- Eat less salt
- Eat more fibre
- Reduce alcohol consumption

By using a smaller plate and eating only when you are physically hungry, you will reduce these automatically. However, if you want to become more conscious of how much you should be eating, the following table will provide you with the recommended guidelines.

Fat	Amount of fat per 100g		
	A LOT	MODERATE	LITTLE
	20g or more	3-20g or more or	3g or less or
	6g of saturates or more	1-5g of saturates	1g of saturates or less
Sugar	Amount of sugar per 100g		
	A LOT	MODERATE	LITTLE
	10g or more	3-10g or more	3g or less
SALT	Amount of salt per 100g		
	A LOT	MODERATE	LITTLE
	1.5g or more or 0.6g sodium	0.3-1.5g or more or 0.1-0.6g sodium	0.3g or less or 0.1g sodium
FIBRE	Amount of fibre per 100g		
	A LOT	MODERATE	LITTLE
	6g or more	3-6g or more	3g or less

WHAT ABOUT CARBS?

Carbohydrates are a source of energy. When eaten, the body converts most carbohydrates into glucose (sugar), which is used to fuel cells such as those of the brain and muscles.

Carbohydrates are one of three macronutrients found in food (nutrients that form a large part of our diet) – the others being fat and protein. Hardly any foods contain only one nutrient and most are a combination of carbohydrates, fats and proteins in varying amounts. There are three different types of carbohydrate: sugar, starch and fibre.

- Sugar is found naturally in some foods, including fruit, honey, fruit juices, milk (lactose) and vegetables. Other forms of sugar (for example table sugar) can be added to food and drink such as sweets, chocolates, biscuits and soft drinks during manufacture, or added when cooking or baking at home. Remember: sugar is a carbohydrate but not all carbs are sugars.

- Starch, made up of many sugar units bonded

together is found in foods that come from plants. Starchy foods, such as bread, rice, potatoes and pasta, provide a slow and steady release of energy throughout the day.

- Fibre is mainly found in foods that come from plants. Fibre helps keep our bowels healthy and some types of fibre may help lower cholesterol. Research shows diets high in fibre are associated with a lower risk of cardiovascular disease, type 2 diabetes and bowel cancer. Good sources of fibre include vegetables with skins on, wholegrain bread, wholewheat pasta and pulses (beans and lentils).

Carbs should be the body's main source of energy in a healthy balanced diet. Carbs are broken down into glucose (sugar) before being absorbed into the bloodstream. From there, the glucose enters the body's cells with the help of insulin. Glucose is used by your body for energy and fuels all of your activities, whether going for a run or breathing. Unused glucose can be converted to glycogen found in the liver and muscles. If unused, glucose can be converted to fat, for long-term storage of energy.

Using the healthy portion plate, eating only when you are hungry and stopping when you are satisfied will as a matter of course reduce your carb intake.

Remember: If you eat more carbs than your body can convert into energy, the extra will be stored as fat and therefore, your weight will increase. Eating less than your body can convert into energy means that once your body has used the energy from the carbs, it will then start to burn body fat.

IT'S DO IT O'CLOCK

- Recognise the differences between hunger and thirst.

- If you are not sure, have a glass of water and leave it half an hour BEFORE eating. Then, if the feeling is still there, and it's genuine hunger - eat.

- Increase your water intake.

- Always use a small plate – no larger than 7 inches (18cm) in diameter, excluding the lip.

- Always leave some food on your plate.

- If you want pudding, leave a similar amount of food from your main course on your plate.

- If you want more than one course, eat a small amount of each – not everything on each plate. Your health and reaching your goal is far more important than sabotaging your results.

CHAPTER 7

PRINCIPLE 6

HOW TO EAT

Time to Get Real!...the worst time to zone out is when you are actually eating.

Changing your eating habits means doing things differently – it means becoming more conscious of what you are doing.

When you zone out and are more interested in what's on the TV, or computer screen, or when reading, etc., there is a real danger that you go from starving to stuffed without any knowledge of how you got there.

Eating s-l-o-w-l-y (which means putting your knife and fork down while you actually CHEW the food in your mouth), instead of having the next forkful ready and poised to go in your mouth before you have even swallowed the last one and paying attention to eating (rather than to the TV etc) allows you to hear the signal from your stomach to your brain that says 'I've had enough'.

Remember: It takes 20 minutes for the stomach to communicate with the brain that it's had enough. Eating quickly, not chewing your food adequately and zoning out means you miss this vital signal.

Also, not chewing your food adequately fills up your stomach, it can make you feel bloated and it exacerbates issues like IBS (Irritable Bowel Syndrome). Aim to chew the food in your mouth until it resembles mush.

WHEN DO YOU EAT YOUR FAVOURITE THINGS?

When I ask my clients to talk me through how they eat a plate of food, 99% of them have said that they leave their favourite thing until last. They leave it until last as a reward for eating everything else, however, if you leave it until last, you are probably already full and are, therefore, about to force down something you have said is your favourite thing. In reality, if you are already full when you get to this, how much are you really going to enjoy it? EAT IT FIRST!

ARRGGHH...MY WEIGHT HAS PLATEAUD

There will be times between now and reaching your goal weight when your weight plateaus – this is normal.

If you shed the excess weight by eating a certain portion size and then you hit a plateau where you stop releasing the excess weight, you need to eat less to break out of the plateau because it takes less energy/calories to move a lighter body after you have released excess weight.

Reduce your portion size to break out of the plateau and continue towards your goal weight.

Continue to keep your food diary so you know how much less to eat if/when you hit another plateau.

IT'S DO IT O'CLOCK

- Eat slowly.

- Eat consciously (pay attention only to eating and not to any external stimuli).

- STOP eating as soon as you are satisfied (not when you are full).

- Eat your favourite thing first.

- When you hit a plateau, reduce your portion sizes.

CHAPTER 8

PRINCIPLE 7

REWARDING YOURSELF

Time to Get Real!...food is not a reward.

You've made progress towards reaching your goal weight, or you've reached a milestone...now what?

A significant number of my clients have talked about rewarding themselves at the end of the week, at the end of the month, when they have had some success, reached a milestone or reached their goal. The rewards they talk about are usually a takeaway, a meal out, chocolate or cake, etc.

WHY?

Why would you 'reward' yourself with the one thing that has made you unhappy for so long?

Is it really a reward, or it is more of a punishment?

Remember: Food is fuel, not a reward.

Decide now to find a more appropriate way of rewarding yourself for your achievement – a way that doesn't involve something that has made you unhappy.

Remember: eating more than you need at times you don't need it has led you to being a weight you are unhappy with.

LICENSING EFFECTS

The Licensing Effect is the natural human tendency to balance things out and often this begins in childhood. How many of us were brought up with such patterns as: you can go out and play after your have tidied your room, you can watch TV after you have done your homework, and you can only have your pudding if you eat all of your dinner first.

In other words, we are used to getting something good (a reward) if we do 'the right thing'. The problem happens when this reward is unhealthy and if the 'good' isn't sufficiently compensatory, for example, you've had a good day in terms of your eating habits and feel licensed to overeat in the evening.

In what ways do the Licensing Effects take place in your life?

LANGUAGE MATTERS

Remember: we search for that which we have lost, so choose another way of communicating both to yourself and to others your results and achievements. For example, instead of saying 'I have lost X pounds/kilograms/stones', say 'I have shed/released/got rid of X pounds/kilograms/stones'.

IT'S DO IT O'CLOCK

- Remember food is not a reward. Reward yourself in more appropriate and effective ways – ways that support you achieving your goal weight.

- Beware of the Licensing Effects in your life.

Final reminder:

Remember: Nothing you eat or drink will EVER taste as good as the feeling of you being at your goal weight.

I'd love to hear how you are getting on.

Keep in touch!

You can email me:

debbie@debbieholden.com

To your success,
Debbie x

For more information about Debbie and her
Programmes, go to:

www.debbieholden.com
www.facebook.com/GetSlimforLife

29245847R00066

Printed in Great Britain
by Amazon